Fatty Liver Solution

A Beginner's Quick Start Guide on Naturally Managing Fatty Liver Disease Through Nutrition

JEFFREY WINZANT

Disclaimer

By reading this disclaimer, you are accepting the terms of the disclaimer in full. If you disagree with this disclaimer, please do not read the guide.

All of the content within this guide is provided for informational and educational purposes only, and should not be accepted as independent medical or other professional advice. The author is not a doctor, physician, nurse, mental health provider, or registered nutritionist/dietician. Therefore, using and reading this guide does not establish any form of a physician-patient relationship.

Always consult with a physician or another qualified health provider with any issues or questions you might have regarding any sort of medical condition. Do not ever disregard any qualified professional medical advice or delay seeking that advice because of anything you have read in this guide. The information in this guide is not intended to be any sort of medical advice and should not be used in lieu of any medical advice by a licensed and qualified medical professional.

The information in this guide has been compiled from a variety of known sources. However, the author cannot attest to or guarantee the accuracy of each source and thus should not be held liable for any errors or omissions.

Introduction

Fatty liver, also known as hepatic steatosis, is a condition that currently affects almost a third of the US population. There are two categories, non-alcoholic fatty liver and alcoholic fatty liver diseases, so when you make poor choices when it comes to consuming unhealthy food, drinking excessive alcohol, and living a sedentary routine, you may end up having fatty liver. Left unchecked, fatty liver can cause damage to the liver and lead to serious medical conditions such as liver fibrosis or scarring, and cirrhosis, which can be fatal.

Usually, the build-up of fat in the liver greatly affects its function in the body, mainly to process nutrients and filter unnecessary substances from food that the body doesn't need. When the liver can't function properly, it leads to serious conditions, not only affecting the liver but as well as the rest of the body.

As of this writing, there are no FDA-approved medications for the direct treatment of fatty liver. Fortunately, and if diagnosed early, this condition is easily reversible by making changes in the patient's diet and lifestyle. Following important changes in your diet and lifestyle will definitely help improve your health and your body.

This guide is great for people diagnosed with fatty liver and who would like to change their diet to a healthier one. This also provides recipe samples and meal plan samples to help you adjust your eating habits and improve your lifestyle to best support your body. There is also additional information on foods you can include in your diet and how it helps your body.

Here are some other things you can expect from reading this guide:

- Brief introduction on the condition
- Information about the Fatty Liver Diet
- How to maintain the diet
- Sample recipes that are fatty liver-friendly
- Lifestyle changes tips to follow for patients

Table of Contents

ALL ABOUT THE FATTY LIVER

From its name alone, the fatty liver condition refers to when fat starts to build up in the liver. Health professionals also call it hepatic steatosis. Take note though, this condition only refers to when the fat buildup is excessive because having a smaller amount of fat in the liver is normal.

The liver is the human body's second-largest organ. Its basic function is to assist in the processing and storing of nutrients from food and drinks and also filtering out harmful substances from the blood. In addition, the liver is also responsible for the metabolism of medicines, important clotting factors, and the production of glucose.

Too much fat in the liver can cause it to become inflamed. This can damage the liver and eventually cause irreversible damage or scarring and in severe cases, death since as some sources claim, the liver is the greatest immune defense of the body; once it fails, all else follows.

If a person who drinks too much alcohol develops fatty liver, the condition is called alcoholic fatty liver or AFLD.

If a person who doesn't drink alcohol is diagnosed with the disease, it's called non-alcoholic fatty liver or NAFLD.

Currently, 25 to 30% of people in Europe and the United States are suffering from NAFLD according to a report released by researchers from the World Journal of Gastroenterology.

What Are the Symptoms?

In most cases, fatty liver is asymptomatic which means there are no noticeable symptoms--- which may be deemed as usual symptoms of normal illnesses.

To be more specific, alcoholic fatty liver may also cause:

- Nausea
- Fever
- Jaundice; and
- Vomiting

Below are some symptoms that may be experienced by people with nonalcoholic fatty liver:

- Unexplained weight loss
- Jaundice
- Decreased appetite
- Swollen legs
- Itchy skin

In general, patients may initially experience general exhaustion or feel pain and discomfort in the upper right side of the abdomen.

When fatty liver is left unchecked, a person suffering from it can develop complications, one of which is liver scarring. This condition is called fibrosis (stage 2 liver disease) and if it gets worse, it can lead to liver cirrhosis (stage 3 liver disease), a potentially deadly medical condition.

Some symptoms of liver cirrhosis include:

- Significant weight loss
- Loss of appetite
- Fatigue
- Weakness
- Itchy skin
- Yellow eyes and skin
- Nosebleeds
- Abdominal pain and swelling
- Swelling legs
- Confusion
- Enlargement of the breast in men

What Causes Fatty Liver?

Fatty liver occurs when the body is producing too much fat and it isn't being metabolized efficiently or fast enough. The excess fat is then stored in the liver where it can accumulate and cause the disease.

There are a variety of factors that can cause this fat build-up. As previously mentioned, drinking too much alcohol can cause AFLD, which is usually the initial stage of liver diseases that are associated with alcohol consumption.

But for people who drink alcohol in moderation or those that totally abstain from it and still develop NAFLD, the cause is less clear.

One or a few of these factors are considered to be potential causes:

- High blood sugar or diabetes
- Obesity
- Resistance to insulin
- High-fat levels in the blood, especially triglycerides

The following can also cause NAFLD but they're less common:

- Rapid weight loss
- Pregnancy
- Infections like hepatitis C
- Side effects due to certain medications which include tamoxifen, methotrexate, valproic acid, and amiodarone.
- Exposure to some toxins

Certain human genes have also been found to increase the risks of having NAFLD.

How Is Fatty Liver Diagnosed?

Diagnosis of the fatty liver includes gathering the patient's medical history, conducting a physical exam, and doing one or more of the following tests:

- Blood test for elevated liver enzymes
- Imaging tests such MRI, CT scan, and ultrasound

-   Liver biopsy

Fatty Liver Treatment

There are currently no approved medications for the treatment of fatty liver. But, in more severe cases of fatty liver wherein patients already have compromised airways, brain damage, and impaired swallowing reflexes, dietary intervention/ management through oral or tube feeding is made under the supervision of a dietitian and a doctor. The diet consists of complex carbohydrates, fats, and proteins in liquid form to give proper nutrition to the patient.

Fortunately, fatty liver is reversible in many cases and is easily accomplished by lifestyle changes like losing excess weight, avoiding or limiting alcohol, and making changes to the patient's diet.

THE FATTY LIVER DIET

One of the most effective approaches to fatty liver is through losing excess body fat. Health experts agree that 70% of weight loss is due to diet.

Although there are no FDA-approved drugs for fatty liver yet, doctors agree that losing around 10% of a person's body weight is a good start, especially for patients who are obese.

NAFLD has been found most common in patients who live a sedentary lifestyle and those who consume mainly highly-processed foods.

Basic Components of the Fatty Liver Diet

A diet plan for people who have fatty liver should include the following:

- Lots of vegetables and fruits
- High-fiber foods like whole grains and legumes
- Reduced consumption of salt, sugar, refined carbohydrates, trans fat, and saturated fat

Basically, the patient should undergo a reduced-calorie, low-fat diet to help in losing the excess weight.

Foods to Include in a Fatty Liver Diet Plan

- **Greens.** In a study, broccoli has been found to be effective in helping prevent fat building in the livers of mice. Consuming more green vegetables like Brussels sprouts, spinach, and kale might also help with weight loss. There are a lot of vegetarian recipes that are full of flavor but low in calories.
- **Coffee.** Research has shown that those with fatty liver who also drink coffee are less susceptible to liver damage than those who don't. It's thought that the caffeine in this beverage reduces the levels of abnormal liver enzymes for those people that have high risks for liver diseases.
- **Fish.** Especially the fatty ones such as sardines, salmon, trout, and tuna, contain significant amounts of healthy omega-3 fatty acids. Omega-3 fatty acids have been found to help in improving fat levels in the liver and significantly reduce inflammation.
- **Tofu.** Soybeans have high protein content. Tofu is a soy product that has high protein content but a very low fat amount. A study made on rats by the University of Illinois showed that soy protein reduces liver fat buildup.
- **Walnuts.** These contain high amounts of omega-3 fatty acids which, as previously discussed, have shown to be beneficial in improving the liver function for patients diagnosed with fatty liver.
- **Oatmeal.** Carbohydrates consumed by patients with fatty liver should come from whole grains like oatmeal. Complex carbohydrates release a steady

amount of energy and the fiber content satiates which is important in weight maintenance.

- **Low-fat dairy.** Whey protein might be able to help in protecting the liver from damage and this is important for those with fatty liver. Milk and other dairy products have high whey protein content but it's recommended for those with reduced fat content.
- **Avocado.** It might be high in fat content but these are the healthy ones. Research suggests that healthy fats and certain chemicals found in avocados can slow down liver damage. Avocados are also fiber-rich which helps in weight control.
- **Olive oil.** It's one of the healthiest and more readily available oils on the market. Olive oil is rich in omega-3 fatty acids and is much healthier when used for food preparation compared to shortening, butter, or margarine. Research shows that it can lower the number of liver enzymes and also help control weight.
- Sunflower seeds. The vitamin E content of the nutty-tasting sunflower seeds can protect the liver from damage due to its antioxidant properties.
- **Green tea.** From aiding with sleep to lowering cholesterol, green tea has shown many medical and health benefits. Initial studies show that green tea helps by interfering with fat absorption. It might also help with improving liver function and reducing fat storage in the organ.
- **Garlic.** It doesn't just add a lot of flavor and aroma to food but garlic powder supplements are also showing potential in the reduction of excess body weight for people with fatty liver.

- **Healthy fats.** Fat is still needed even in people prone to fatty liver disease. Choosing healthy fats such as fish oil, nuts, vegetable oils, and omega-3 fatty acids is smarter since they are unsaturated and do not stay in the liver.

Foods to Avoid

The following foods should be avoided or consumption limited for patients with fatty liver. These contribute to increased blood sugar levels and weight gain which should be avoided when treating the disease.

- **Alcohol.** It's not only the major cause of the disease but also for other organ diseases.
- **Fried food.** These are soaked in saturated fat and generally high in calories.
- **Added sugar.** Sugary foods such as cookies, candies, fruit juices, and soda should be avoided. High levels of sugar in the blood can increase liver fat buildup.
- **Pasta, rice, and bread.** Especially the white ones because the flour used has been highly processed. These can raise blood sugar levels. Opt for brown rice and whole wheat bread and pasta as these have higher fiber content that can help eliminate fat and unhealthy cholesterol from the body.
- **Salt.** Salt is linked to water retention and also causes fat buildup and high blood pressure but it's an essential ingredient of most foods. Limit consumption to no more than 1.5 grams per day.
- **Red meat.** Avoid deli meats and beef because these have high saturated fat content.

STEPS IN MAINTAINING A FATTY LIVER DIET

Treating fatty liver with food is basically eating healthy. Here are some tips to consider for people with this condition

Eating Regular Meals

Eating regularly makes controlling appetite easier because it can reduce cravings and helps in planning healthy meals. Aim to have 3 major meals per day.

Follow the Mediterranean Diet Pyramid

Fruits and vegetables, legumes, seeds, nuts, cereals, and whole grain bread should take up most of the calories the patient consumes. Proteins should come from lean sources like fish, chicken breasts, and eggs. Low-fat dairy also provides additional protein, calcium, and other nutrients.

When the body gets enough nutrition coming from these food groups, craving for high sugar and high fat is greatly reduced.

Choose Healthier Drinks

Water is still the best beverage, especially for those people who are trying to lose weight. It contains zero calories and drinking a glass before a meal reduces food intake. Avoid drinks with too much sugar like juices, sports drinks, cordials, and sodas. Also, avoid alcohol as it can worsen fatty liver. Not only does it give more work for the liver, when alcohol calories don't get burned, but they are also stored as fat in other parts of the body as well.

Reduce Portion Sizes

Replace that dinner plate with a salad plate. Studies show that the bigger the plate, the more food is consumed. Use smaller bowls and plates to reduce calorie intake.

Choose Healthier Alternatives

Eat more vegetables, fruits, legumes, wholegrain, high-fiber cereals, and bread. These satiate faster and longer but with fewer calories. In cooking, you can opt to skip table salt or sugar and lean into using spices. These improve the meal flavors, and at the same time, have better effects on health.

Here are examples of replacing food choices with better alternatives:

- Instead of a 1/3 bowl of muesli, eat a 2/3 bowl of oats
- Instead of a glass of fruit drink, eat 3 pieces of fruits
- Instead of 40 grams of chocolate, eat 2 slices multigrain bread

Both choices have the same calorie content but the latter is more filling than the former.

Plan Ahead

Planning meals ahead can help limit instances of impulse eating, the temptation of grabbing a takeaway, and other spur-of-the-moment food choices. Prepare a meal plan for the whole week and shop for the ingredients in the supermarket. Cooking meals and storing them in the refrigerator or freezer also helps a lot in controlling calorie intake. In addition, avoid going to the groceries when hungry to avoid impulsive, unhealthy buys.

DIET PLAN AND SAMPLE RECIPES FOR FATTY LIVER PATIENTS

Sample Meal Plan

A typical meal plan for a patient with fatty liver might look like this:

Meal	Menu
Breakfast	- Hot oatmeal (8 oz.), mixed with almond butter (2 tsp.) and sliced banana (1 pc.) - Coffee with skim or low-fat milk (1 cup)
Lunch	- Salad greens with olive oil and balsamic vinegar dressing - Grilled chicken, 3 oz. - Baked small potato - Cooked carrots or broccoli, 1 cup - Apple, 1 pc. - Milk, 1 glass
Snack	- Raw veggies with 2 tbsp. of hummus or sliced apples with 1 tbsp. peanut butter
Dinner	- Mixed-bean salad, small - Grilled salmon, 3 oz. - Cooked broccoli, 1 cup - Whole-grain roll, 1 pc - Mixed berries, 1 cup - Milk, 1 glass

Another sample meal plan for a whole day:

Meal	Menu
Breakfast	- High-fiber cereal with low-fat milk or multigrain bread (2 slices) with tomato / baked beans / peanut butter / mushrooms / cottage cheese - Fruit, 1 pc. - Water
Morning Tea	- Fruit (1 pc) / Greek yogurt (100 – 200 g) / oatmeal biscuits (2 pcs.) / fruit bread (1 thin slice) / grainy crackers with tomato and cottage cheese (2 pcs.) / raw nuts (5 to 6 pcs.)
Lunch	- 1 wrap / 1 bread roll / multigrain bread (2 slices) - Green salad with low-fat cheese / chicken / salmon / tuna - Water
Afternoon Tea	- Fruit (1 pc) / Greek yogurt (100 – 200 g) / oatmeal biscuits (2 pcs.) / fruit bread (1 thin slice) / grainy crackers with tomato and cottage cheese (2 pcs.) / raw nuts (5 to 6 pcs.)
Dinner	- 120 g lean chicken / eggs / chicken / legumes - Vegetables (zucchini / spinach / peas / cauliflower / carrots / cabbage / broccoli / beans - Whole wheat pasta (1 cup) / Brown rice (2/3 cup) / sweet potato (1/2 cup) / medium potato (1 pc.) - Water

Just because you're going low-calorie does not mean you have to put up with bland food. There are ways to add flavor to any food without putting in too much salt or sugar. Here

are some sample recipes that are low in calorie content but big
in flavor.

Lemon-Baked Salmon

Ingredients:

- 2 pcs. lemons, thinly sliced
- 3 lbs. salmon filet
- kosher salt
- black pepper, freshly ground
- 6 tbsp. butter, melted, 6 tbsp.
- 2 tbsp. honey
- 3 cloves garlic, minced
- 1 tsp. thyme leaves, chopped
- 1 tsp. dried oregano
- fresh parsley, chopped, for garnish

Instructions:

1. Preheat the oven to 350°F.
2. Line a rimmed baking sheet with foil. Grease with cooking oil spray.
3. Lay lemon slices on the center of the foil.
4. Season salmon filets on both sides with kosher salt and freshly ground black pepper.

5. Place the filet on top of the lemon slices.
6. Whisk together oregano, thyme, garlic, honey, and butter in a small bowl.
7. Pour the mixture over the salmon filet.
8. Fold the foil up and around the salmon to form a packet.
9. Bake for 25 minutes or until the salmon is cooked through.
10. Switch to broil and continue cooking for 2 more minutes.
11. Garnish with chopped fresh parsley and serve hot.

Grilled Chicken Breast

Ingredients:

- 4 pcs. skinless, boneless, chicken breasts
- 1 tbsp. sugar
- 1 tsp. garlic powder
- 2 tbsp. Italian seasoning
- 1 tbsp. pepper
- 1 tbsp. salt
- 2 tbsp. lemon juice
- 3 tbsp. Worcestershire sauce
- 2 tbsp. Dijon mustard
- 1/4 cup cider vinegar
- 1/3 cup olive oil

Instructions:

1. Combine all of the ingredients in a Ziploc bag or large bowl. Massage or toss until well combined.

2. Marinade the chicken breasts for at least 30 minutes. You can also refrigerate for up to 4 hours.
3. Preheat the grill to medium to medium-high heat.
4. Place marinated chicken breasts on the grill and cook for 7 to 8 minutes.
5. Flip them over and cook for another 7 to 8 minutes. The internal temperature of the chicken should be 165 degrees when checked with a meat thermometer.
6. Take the chicken off the grill and place it on a serving plate.
7. Allow the chicken to rest for 3 to 5 minutes before slicing and serving.

Mixed Bean Salad

Ingredients:

- 400 g. tin can mixed bean salad, drained and rinsed
- 2 stalks spring onions, finely chopped
- 2 sticks celery, thinly sliced
- 1 pc. large tomato, deseeded and finely diced
- salt
- freshly ground black pepper

For the dressing:

- 3 tbsp. olive oil
- 1 tbsp. white wine vinegar
- 1 tsp. sugar
- 2 tsp. Dijon mustard
- 1 tbsp. fresh tarragon, chopped

- 1 tbsp. fresh parsley, chopped

Instructions:

1. Put mixed beans, spring onions, celery, and tomato in a salad bowl.
2. Add salt and pepper to taste. Mix well.
3. In a separate bowl, mix the ingredients for the dressing until well combined.
4. Pour the dressing on the salad and toss well.
5. Serve immediately.

Liver Detox Smoothie

Ingredients:

- 1-inch fresh turmeric
- 1/2 cup raw beets, shredded
- 1 cup raw spinach leaves
- 1/2 cup fresh apple or unsweetened apple sauce
- 1 cup unsweetened almond milk, coconut water, or choice milk
- lemon juice from a half or a full lemon

Instructions:

1. Chop roughly the apple and turmeric.
2. Shred the beets using a cheese grater.
3. Put all the ingredients in a blender.
4. Blend high until they are completely smooth.

Oatmeal Almond Cookies

Ingredients:

- 3/4 cup almond flour
- 1/2 tsp. cinnamon
- cranberries, dried and chopped into smaller bits
- 3/4 cup gluten-free rolled oats
- 1/4 cup maple syrup
- a pinch of salt
- optional: 2 tbsp. cacao nibs

Instructions:

1. Preheat your oven to 350° Fahrenheit.
2. Put the oats in the food processor, blender, or spice grinder and pulse until the oats are already ground into a meal. Put the ground oats in a bowl. Add the cinnamon, almond flour, and salt. Mix the ingredients well.
3. Pour the coconut oil into the bowl. Smash lightly into the flour using the back of a spoon. Put in the maple syrup, and mix it well.
4. Stir the cranberries and cacao nibs in.
5. Line the prepared baking sheet with Silpat or parchment paper. To scoop the cookies onto the baking sheet, use a 1/4 measuring cup and flatten the cookies until they are almost half-inch thick.
6. Bake the cookies for fifteen minutes.

HOW TO GET USED TO THE FATTY LIVER DIET

It may be easy to read, think, and try changing your lifestyle in order to be healthy. But, it is a given fact that changing one's lifestyle is not easy to do and maintain. So, the following are tips on how to maintain the diet and achieve your goal of a healthier liver.

Take it slowly. Every process is composed of a series of steps. And these steps should be taken seriously as this will lead you to the next. Thus, doing this diet is not an overnight thing. You can first start making healthier choices. Then, follow it up with regular exercise if you have already adapted to doing a healthier diet. Do not worry about doing it all together as this will only stress you and may prevent you from continuing to do so.

Trust the process. As mentioned in the previous tip, dieting is not an overnight thing. So, do not expect to see changes immediately. The fat in your liver took time to build up, thus it will also require time, discipline, and consistency in order to go back to normal. Just follow what is suggested and stick to it.

Be consistent. Losing weight is a step toward having a healthier liver. But it doesn't mean that you lose weight, you

also lose the fat in your liver. So, be happy when there are positive changes that are happening in your body. It means that you are already doing a great job. But what makes the job you are doing even better is if you continue to do what you have started.

Choose foods and activities that are comfortable for you. Even though there are suggested food items in this book, it doesn't mean that your options are limited to those. You can ask your doctor or dietitian, or do your research on similar food items that provide the same function and nutrient content. If you do not like almonds, you can opt for hazelnuts. If you do not like beets, you may try carrots. As long as it offers the same function, do as you please. Nothing's more discouraging if you are forced to eat what you don't like. It's the same with activities. If you are more comfortable working out in your home, then you can opt to do cardio exercises or aerobics in place instead of running, cycling, or running which requires you to go to places. It's your diet, so it's your choice.

Think about the long-term benefits. Are you afraid of the consequences which may be brought by fatty liver disease? Take this as a motivation to start or continue this diet. Would you rather pay thousands of bucks (or more) for expensive maintenance, regular hospital visits, and the worst-case--- hospitalization? Or would you rather eat healthier, exercise regularly, and avoid food that may affect your liver? You choose.

LIFESTYLE CHANGES

Treating fatty liver disease and reversing the damage is all about lowering body weight. A 10 percent reduction in excess weight is enough to improve enzyme levels in the liver according to doctors.

Aside from the diet, another recommendation from doctors is for those with the fatty liver to make a change in their lifestyles. Most patients diagnosed with NAFLD live a sedentary life with very little to no physical activity.

Here are some changes the patient should make to improve liver health.

Avoid Alcohol

This can't be reiterated enough. The liver goes through a lot of stress during alcohol consumption since it is the one breaking down alcohol calories, not the stomach. Imagine that stress on an already diseased liver.

Lose Weight

But not rapidly. Losing 1 to 2 pounds per week should be the goal. And this may be done by deducting 500 kilocalories from your daily food intake. That means setting aside two

muffins, one large fries, or almost a quarter pounder, and a bottle of soda every day. Shedding off those extra pounds lowers inflammation and prevents further injury to the liver.

Exercise

Aerobic has shown to be most effective in cutting fat levels in the liver. Walk, jog, or run regularly. Physical exercise also lowers inflammation. Exercise at least 3 times a week.

Manage Diabetes

For patients who are also suffering from diabetes, they should consult their doctor for proper management. The inability of the body to process sugar properly due to diabetes puts additional stress on the liver.

Lower Cholesterol Levels

Keep triglycerides and cholesterol levels down. This can be done through medication or eating a plant-based diet, and regular exercise. In addition, fiber-rich foods such as beans, oatmeal, nuts, fruits, and vegetables, help in reducing bad cholesterol levels.

Benefits of the Fatty Liver Diet Plan

No more nasty symptoms. Although fatty liver disease may show little to no distinctive symptoms. Most symptoms such as confusion, fatigue, fever, abdominal pain, loss of appetite, and physical weakness are a hassle for your everyday life. So, doing the diet may help alleviate these symptoms since the diet mostly consists of healthier food options.

Less risk for other diseases. Experts say that fatty liver disease is associated with several diseases such as diabetes, obesity, protein-energy malnutrition, hypertension, and hyper cholesterol. Since the diet not only involves the consumption of healthy foods but also recommendations to do regular exercise, the risk of the mentioned diseases may also be lessened. It's like hitting a ton of birds with one stone.

Worry-free life. Once you have gotten rid of the fatty liver, you have already lessened your risk for lifestyle diseases that may induce other complications. Thus, doing this diet will make you get rid of the unfavorable fatty liver disease symptoms and the difficulty in doing normal daily physical activities. It also strengthens your immune system because the diet is high in vitamins and minerals that help keep the body and its organs functioning well.

Green Smoothie

Ingredients:

- 6 dandelion greens, chopped
- 4 kale leaves, stems removed, chopped
- 1 Meyer or organic lemon, peeled and sliced into chunks
- 1 Fuji apple, cut into chunks
- 2 cups filtered water
- Optional: 1 small banana, peeled and sliced
- Optional: 1 tsp. grated ginger

Instructions:

1. Place all ingredients into a blender
2. Blend on high speed for 1-2 minutes
3. Add more water if necessary.
4. Serve and enjoy.

Detox Juice

Ingredients:

- 1 beet, scrubbed
- 1 apple
- 1 lemon, peeled
- 1 cucumber, peeled
- one handful of dandelion greens, washed

Instruction:

1. Juice everything and stir well.

Lentil Soup

Ingredients:

- 1 tbsp. avocado oil
- 1 cup onion, diced
- 1/2 cup carrot, diced
- 1/2 cup celery, diced
- 4 cups vegetable or chicken broth
- 1 cup dried red lentils, well rinsed
- 1/4 tsp dried thyme
- 1/2 cup fresh flat-leaf parsley, chopped
- salt and pepper, to taste

Instructions:

1. Sauté carrot, celery and onion in a large saucepan over medium heat. Do so until they are soft.
2. Pour in the broth with lentils and thyme and wait to boil.

3. Lower the heat. Cover and leave to simmer until lentils are soft, about 20 minutes.
4. Transfer soup to a blender.
5. Set the blender on high. Purée the soup until it's creamy.
6. If it's too thick, pour in a cup of water.
7. Add salt and pepper to taste.
8. Return to the saucepan to reheat if necessary.
9. Ladle into bowls and garnish with parsley.
10. Serve and enjoy while hot.

Ragi Oat Crackers with Cucumber Dip

Ingredients:

- 1/2 cup ragi flour, also called nachni flour or red millet flour
- 2 tsp. olive oil
- 1/2 cup whole-wheat flour
- 1/4 cup rolled oats, quick cooking
- 1/2 tsp. garlic paste
- 1/2 tsp. green chili paste
- salt, to taste

Cucumber dip:

- 1 cup low-fat hung curd, whisked
- 1/2 cup cucumber, grated
- 2 tbsp. coriander, chopped finely
- 2 tbsp. mint leaves, chopped finely

- 1/4 tsp. cumin seeds powder
- 1/4 tsp. garlic paste
- salt, to taste

To make the ragi oat crackers:

1. Combine ingredients in a deep bowl and knead into a stiff dough using enough water.
2. Divide dough into 2 equal portions.
3. Roll out a portion into a 200 mm diameter circle. Don't use flour for rolling.
4. Prick dough all over using a fork.
5. Cut into small square pieces, approximately 12 pieces.
6. Repeat steps 3 and 4 to make 12 more pieces using the other dough portion.
7. Preheat the oven to 360°F.
8. Arrange square dough on a greased baking tray.
9. Bake for about 12 minutes. Turn them on the other side and bake again until crispy on both sides.
10. Keep aside to cool slightly.
11. Store in an airtight container.

To make the cucumber dip:

1. Mix ingredients in a bowl.
2. Serve with the ragi oat crackers and enjoy.

Veggies and Chicken Skillet

Ingredients:

- 1/4 cup all-purpose flour

- 2 oz. baby carrots
- 1 cup cherry tomatoes
- finely chopped medium onion, 1 piece
- fresh sliced cremini mushroom, 7 oz
- ground pepper
- 2 tbsp. olive oil
- salt
- 14 oz. chicken breasts, skinless and boneless
- 1 cup vegetable or chicken stock
- optional: fresh parsley, for garnish

Instruction:

1. Pound chicken breasts until they are one inch thick.
2. Put flour on a shallow plate. Add the salt and pepper to the plate and then mix.
3. Use this mixture to dredge the chicken breasts. Set aside.
4. Heat olive oil in a large skillet.
5. Add the chicken breasts. Cook them until they start to look brown. Set aside on a plate.
6. In the same skillet pan, add the carrots, mushrooms, and onion.
7. Sauté the ingredients for around 4-5 minutes.
8. Add stock to cover up the chicken. Let the stock come to a boil.
9. Simmer with the lid on for 15-20 minutes
10. Add the cherry tomatoes and simmer. Wait until they have softened.
11. To garnish, just top the veggies and chicken skillet with the finely chopped fresh parsley.
12. Serve and enjoy hot.

Quinoa Tacos

Ingredients:

Quinoa:

- 1 cup white, tricolor, or red quinoa, rinsed well
- 1 cup vegetable broth or stock
- 3/4 cup water

Seasoning:

- 1/2 cup salsa with slightly chunky bits
- 1 tbsp. nutritional yeast
- 2 tsp. ground cumin
- 2 tsp. ground chili powder
- 1/2 tsp. garlic powder
- 1/2 tsp. sea salt
- 1/2 tsp. black pepper
- 1 tbsp. avocado oil or olive oil

Instruction:

1. Heat a medium-sized saucepan over medium heat.
2. Put the quinoa then toast for around 4-5 minutes.
3. Pour water and vegetable broth. Bring it to a boil over medium-high heat.
4. Reduce the heat to low and cook for 15-25 minutes with the lid covered.
5. Fluff up quinoa using a fork.

6. Remove the lid and remove from heat. Leave it to rest for 10 minutes.
7. Preheat your oven to 190°C (375°F) at this point.
8. Add the cooked quinoa into a large mixing bowl. Put the salsa, cumin, nutritional yeast, chili powder, salt, pepper, garlic powder, and oil into the bowl with the cooked quinoa. Toss the ingredients
9. Line a parchment paper or lightly grease a baking sheet. Spread the mixture in the sheet.
10. Bake the mixture for 20-35 minutes.

Avocado, Cucumber, and Tomato Salad

Ingredients:

- 1/4 cup extra-virgin olive oil
- 1 pc. lemon, juiced
- 1/4 tsp. cumin, ground
- salt, to taste
- freshly ground black pepper, to taste
- 3 medium avocados, cubed
- 1-pint cherry tomatoes, halved
- 1 small cucumber, sliced into half-moons
- 1/3 cup corn
- 2 tbsp. cilantro, chopped

Instructions:

1. Combine avocados, cilantro, corn, cucumber, jalapeño, and tomatoes in a large bowl.

2. In a separate small container, whisk together lemon juice, cumin, and oil to make the salad dressing.
3. Season the dressing with salt and pepper.
4. Toss the salad gently while adding the dressing.
5. Serve immediately.

Arugula and Mushroom Salad

Ingredients:

- 5 oz. arugula washed
- 1 lb. fresh mushrooms
- 1/4 tsp. shoyu
- 1/2 red onion
- 1 tbsp. olive oil
- 1 tbsp. mirin

For tofu cheese:

- 1/8 cup umeboshi vinegar
- 1/2 firm tofu

Instructions:

1. In a bowl, add the rinsed tofu. Crumble and pour in vinegar.
2. In a separate bowl add shoyu, red onions, salt, olive oil, and mirin. 3. Mix to combine.
3. Add in the arugula and toss to combine with the dressing.
4. Serve and enjoy.

Tofu Scramble

Ingredients:

- 1 block drained tofu, sliced into an inch
- 2-3 tsp. oil
- 1/2 onion, diced
- salt, to taste
- ground black pepper, to taste
- 2/3 cups salsa
- optional: 2 tsp. nutritional yeast
- optional: 1/3 tsp. turmeric

Instructions:

1. In a large pan, put the oil and sauté the chopped onion.
2. Add the tofu. Pour out oil if needed, and stir frequently.
3. Add the yeast and turmeric. Stir.
4. When the tofu slices are all coated, add the salsa. Stir frequently.
5. Wait for 1 to 2 minutes for it to be cooked. Season with salt and pepper.
6. Serve while warm.

Smoked Salmon and Baked Eggs in Avocado

Ingredients:

- 4 oz. smoked salmon

- 8 eggs
- 4 avocados, halved and deseeded
- fresh dill
- red chili flakes
- salt
- black pepper

Instructions:

1. Preheat the oven to 425°F.
2. In preparing the avocado, make sure that the hole where the seed was can fit an egg. Carve it out more if needed.
3. Place the avocados on a baking sheet.
4. Put smoked salmon strips on each hollow.
5. Crack open an egg in a small bowl. Spoon out the yolk and the white and transfer to the avocado. Carefully eyeball how much egg the avocado can hold.
6. Sprinkle the avocado with salt and pepper.
7. Bake in the oven for about 15-20 minutes.
8. Top with dill and chili flakes upon serving.

Marinated Tuna Steak

Ingredients:

- 4 slices tuna steak
- 1/3 cup soy sauce
- 1 tbsp. cider vinegar
- 3 tbsp. olive oil
- 2 tbsp. parsley, chopped
- 1 tbsp. rosemary, chopped

- 1/2 tsp. oregano, chopped
- 1/8 tsp. garlic powder

Instructions:

1. Put together olive oil, soy sauce, parsley, cider vinegar, rosemary, and oregano in a bowl. Mix well to create a marinade mixture.
2. Using a gallon plastic bag, put tuna steaks and marinade mixture. Allow the mixture to coat the tuna by turning the bag over.
3. Leave inside the refrigerator for 30 minutes.
4. Put a small amount of oil on the grill grate. Cook tuna for about 5 minutes per side.
5. Put some of the remaining marinade mixtures on the tuna every few minutes.

Conclusion

Fatty liver disease is an easily preventable and treatable condition and it doesn't even require expensive medication or treatment methods. The patient just needs to eat a healthy, balanced diet and indulge in exercise to lower body weight and improve liver health.

Avoid consuming highly-processed foods which are usually loaded with salt, sugar, and fats. Instead opt for whole foods, especially fruits and vegetables. Cutting down or completely abstaining from alcohol is also required.

As the saying goes, prevention is always better than the cure and the same applies to fatty liver. Eating healthy and exercising regularly should be a conscious choice. These ensure the protection of not only the liver but the whole body as well.

References and Helpful Links

El-Zayadi, A.-R. (2008). Hepatic steatosis: A benign disease or a silent killer. World Journal of Gastroenterology : WJG, 14(26), 4120–4126. https://doi.org/10.3748/wjg.14.4120.

Everything you need to know about fatty liver. (2021, November 2). Healthline. https://www.healthline.com/health/fatty-liver.

Fatty liver disease highly prevalent in American adults. (2020, August 19). Hep. https://www.hepmag.com/article/fatty-liver-disease-highly-prevalent-american-adults

Fatty liver disease: Risk factors, symptoms, types & prevention. (n.d.). Cleveland Clinic. Retrieved January 14, 2023, from https://my.clevelandclinic.org/health/diseases/15831-fatty-liver-disease.

Fatty liver disease. (n.d.). American Liver Foundation. Retrieved January 14, 2023, from https://liverfoundation.org/about-your-liver/facts-about-liver-disease/fatty-liver-disease/.

What is hepatic steatosis? (2020, August 10). Fatty Liver Disease. https://fattyliverdisease.com/what-is-hepatic-steatosis/.